Guillain-Barré Syndrome:
Through the Eyes of a Mother

Guylaine Barber

Order this book online at www.trafford.com
or email orders@trafford.com

Most Trafford titles are also available at major online book retailers.

Note for Librarians: A cataloguing record for this book is available from Library
and Archives Canada at www.collectionscanada.ca/amicus/index-e.html

Printed in Victoria, BC, Canada.

ISBN: 978-1-4269-1489-8

*Our mission is to efficiently provide the world's finest, most comprehensive book publishing
service, enabling every author to experience success. To find out how to publish your book, your
way, and have it available worldwide, visit us online at www.trafford.com*

Trafford rev. 09/15/09

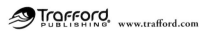

www.trafford.com

North America & international
toll-free: 1 888 232 4444 (USA & Canada)
phone: 250 383 6864 ♦ fax: 812 355 4082

This book is dedicated to the two most important people in my life. My daughter, Cynthia, for her strength and determination to fight this virus, and to my daughter, Sam, for helping me live through a parent's nightmare, dealing with my moods, tears, and understanding that I would have liked to have spent more time with her during that summer of 2006.

CONTENTS

PREFACE

EVERY PARENT HOPES THAT their children will have a wonderful life. That they will grow to be the best they can be. To protect them from the day they are born. To make sure they are properly dressed so they don't catch a cold, to childproof your house when they start crawling, to buy them the best baby shoes so their tiny feet will form properly. You teach them to wash their hands so they won't get sick, you instruct them to look both ways before crossing the street so they won't get hit, you make them wear a helmet when they ride their bike. You teach them all these fundamental things. Then one day some kind of virus comes and quickly you learn that your mommy powers don't work anymore.

I wrote this book to the best of my recollection, to share with others that no matter what cards you are dealt, you can win, one way or another.

CHAPTER 1
THE BEGINNING

"HAWKS UNLEASH HELL," SHOUTED the Henry Street High School women's rugby team. They were pumped to start an all-day tournament so they would be ready for the real big one, LOSSA finals. The sun was shining on this Friday in mid-May in a small suburban town named Whitby, which borders lake Ontario, population of 110,000, when a young woman's dreams were shattered. Senior prom was coming, turning 18 in a few weeks, this beautiful 5-foot-7, 130-pound healthy and competitive rugby player, with brown hair and brown eyes, knew rugby was her game and bruises were her fame. Cynthia only had a bright future to look forward to, college next year, in love, what could be better? Cynthia had met Corey, a baseball player and fellow high school student, with whom she spent most of her time.

Practice every morning, Cynthia would be ready to tackle her next victim on the field, all in good sportsmanship of course. Coach "Puck" encouraged his team of young women to strive for their best, work hard, and be a team. He knew them all by name or almost. On May 16 a few days after the big tournament, Cynthia started experiencing pain from her knees all the way to the end of her toes. An unusual sensation, something hard to describe she would tell me: "It's not a muscle pain Mom, it's like a tingling," along with lower back pain. My first thought was that she must have over done it at the tournament a few days ago and that she would soon recover.

Life went on as usual, and the next day Cynthia returned to school. With the end of the semester approaching, dedication to studies were required to obtain the highest mark possible for College in Cynthia's case and Grade 10 for Sam her sister. Cynthia also needed to make an important decision in the next few days. She struggled when it came to making a decision with what she was going to do for the rest of her life. It was a lot of pressure for a 17-year-old. We talked about it many times. We evaluated what she liked and what she didn't; she spoke to her favourite teacher, her rugby coach and woodshop teacher, to get his advice. Since a young age, Cynthia liked to investigate, take things apart, put them back together, see how they worked, and create unusual things. In Grade 9, duct tape was her thing. Those magic fingers of hers made a duct tape skirt, flip flops, wallet, purse, binders, pens, even a tool belt for her teacher; you name it she made it out of duct tape! That year she was known as the "duct tape girl." Cynthia also loved to work with wood and enjoyed assembling barbecues, bikes, whatever was needed, no instructions required. Finally, after putting all these qualities together, she decided she would apply to George Brown College in Toronto to pursue a career as a home/building inspector, after taking one more semester at high school.

Later that day, Cynthia phoned me at my work, asking my permission for her to leave school early as she wasn't feeling well. She had a rugby practice that afternoon, and I knew she would not miss it unless she was feeling sick. I arrived home that evening to find her lying on the couch still complaining about her legs and back and now feeling nauseated.

By the next morning, she was doubled over the toilet for most of the day. I thought she had the stomach flu, for what else could it be? Lying on the couch again when I got home, Cynthia was for the second day now not feeling well—vomiting, with pain in her legs and back. Corey, her boyfriend, came over after school to comfort her. I decided that we needed to go to the walk-in clinic and see what the doctor had to say, thinking it would be better to be safe than sorry. Off we went, with Cynthia trying not to be sick in the car, while Corey comforted her and I worried as any mother would. Cynthia was examined within a matter of minutes and was diagnosed with tonsillitis. Even though we emphasized to the doctor that her legs and back were very painful, it didn't seem to matter or get through. "Here's a prescription for penicillin," the doctor said. Getting back into the car, Cynthia's first words were, "I'm not taking this, my throat is sore because I've been throwing up all day Mom, not because I have tonsillitis." Cynthia was not a fan of drugs. She didn't believe in smoking or drugs. And the doctor's advice didn't take care of what really was hurting her— her legs and back.

Around 10 that night, we were off for another car ride, this time to Ajax Hospital. The pain was unbearable and she couldn't take it anymore. For my daughter to ask to go to the hospital emergency, I knew she was really hurting. Cynthia and hospital is like cat and water, it doesn't happen very often.

Lots of tears ran down that beautiful face of hers, and I felt so helpless. All I knew to do at this point was to take her where they should have been able to help us. Crying and curled up into a ball, Cynthia waited for her name to be called. During the many hours of waiting to see a doctor, she rocked herself to ease the pain and tried to stay brave. After many hours of waiting, laying on a bed in a small cold room, the doctor casually came in and asked, "So what's wrong with you, why are you crying?" After repeating ourselves for the third time, Cynthia said, "I'm in pain, my lower back is killing me and my legs from my knees to my toes are tingling." Blood tests were done for many different things, such as potassium deficiency, blood count, etc. The results would take another 2½ hours to come back. In the meantime, I was doing my best to rub her back, read to her from an old magazine, rub her forehead, anything to comfort her, but, unfortunately, pain, fatigue, and the fact that she hated hospitals took its toll; all she wanted at this point was to go home.

"Mommy, let's go home," she told me, "I don't want to be here anymore, this was a mistake, take me home pleasssssssse Mommy." Well, that just broke my heart, but since we had waited this long, I thought it was better to stay and hear the test results. Finally, the doctor came to give us his diagnosis. Cynthia sat up to listen but had to rush to the bathroom to throw up. That seemed unusual to me—she had stopped vomiting over five hours ago but now, had started again. They couldn't find anything wrong.

After waiting all this time...no answer. They gave her an injection of Gravol, prescribed a pain killer, an anti-inflammatory, and we were sent home. It was now 3 in the morning on May 19. Here we were, back in the car, driving home, with no more information than when we first started five hours ago. I felt powerless to help my child feel better.

After a few hours of sleep, I went to work as usual. Cynthia was still asleep when I left, and I was hoping that she'd be feeling better by the time I got home that night. Around 10 that morning, Cynthia phoned me. She was a little hungry and I suggested she should try some dry toast. By then I thought that she must have been feeling better since she was starting to get her appetite back. Well I was wrong. By noon, while I was having lunch with a co-worker, my cellphone rang. Cynthia called to tell me that she couldn't go to the washroom, that she really needed to go but couldn't and it was very painful. As a mom, what came to mind was a bladder infection. I left work and arrived home to find Cynthia crying, with pain coming from many different areas of her body.

My friend, Lisa, had come over that afternoon as we had planned to have dinner together. Instead, she offered to drive Cynthia and me to another walk-in clinic. I brought all the medications that Cynthia had been prescribed in the last 48 hours—penicillin, pain killer, and anti-inflammatory. The wait wasn't very long for once. We explained to the doctor the situation, not knowing at the time that this was going to be one of hundreds of times of repeating our story. He asked Cynthia to produce a urine sample, and she replied, "If I could go, I wouldn't be here." He responded, "Oh go on, you go and try." Off she went with this look on her face that she was not impressed. It took her awhile but she came back successful, managing a few trickles. The doctor announced, "You already have what can cure an infection, you have penicillin, that's what you need for an infection. We won't have the results for you until Monday, today being Friday and the lab is closed over the weekend. If there is an infection we'll call you," and that was that.

By that time the pain killers had started to work somewhat; the pain was still there but she could deal with it. That night she started taking the penicillin.

With a hot pack on her lower back, water trickling like when they are little to help them go when you potty train them, and lots of time spent in the bathroom she could go just enough to ease the pain. She did this all night long.

Lisa and I ordered Chinese food that night and Cynthia hung out with us. Sam was out doing what 14-year-old girls do best, hang out with their friends.

On Saturday morning, I had some errands to run so I left the house around 11. Cynthia watched TV, feeling the best she could while she waited for all her meds to kick in. I was gone for a couple of hours when I got a call from her asking me when I would be home. "Very soon, I'm actually on my way home. Everything okay?" I asked. She said, "I just want you to be home with me."

By the time 4 pm came, her health situation had changed. She asked, "Mom, do you hear this?" I stopped and listened to her breathing and it sounded raspy. Right away I asked her, "Do you feel like your throat is closing in?" I thought she might be having an allergic reaction to the penicillin, since she had just started taking it the night before. She said, "No Mommy, it's more like phlegm, a cold I guess."

We spent the night watching TV together. Cynthia started to cough, and as the night went on her cough increased, to the point that it was almost constant. She would fall asleep and wake up from coughing. Here was my daughter laying there sick as a dog, taking all these meds, and there was nothing more I could think to do to help her. I had already taken her to see three doctors. I had researched her different symptoms on the Web, yet she was still feeling terribly sick. I wanted to take her pain away, and just like any other mom, I would have rather been sick than to see my child suffer.

At around 10 that night I got ready for bed and asked Cynthia if she was coming up with me. She replied, "No, I'm more comfortable down here Mom." I said, "Fine, but if you need anything just call for me," and I retired to my bedroom. I must have dozed off but about an hour or so later I awoke to Cynthia's coughing. I decided that she needed to get some rest so I got up, grabbed the cough medicine from the hall closet, went downstairs to the kitchen, and poured a spoonful of medicine for her. I called her to the kitchen to take the meds, but as she made her way to the kitchen, half asleep, she collapsed to the kitchen floor, while she tried to hold on to the counter.

I turned around, dropped the spoon and bottle, and reached to try to soften her fall. First thing I thought of to say was, "Oh my God, you must be so weak because of not eating the last few days." Her eyes looked weird; she was looking at me, but she wasn't. She was so flimsy, her body like rubber. That's when it all started—a journey that seemed to have no end—months of not knowing what was going on, what was happening, or why it was happening to her, to us.

CHAPTER 2
THE CALL

"911, PLEASE STATE YOUR emergency." "My daughter just collapsed on the floor, she's breathing really heavy." "Are her eyes open, can she hear you?" the operator asked. I said, "I think so, Cynthia, Cynthia stay with Mommy, Cynthia can you hear me? Oh my God help me I don't know what to do." The operator ordered, "Stay with her, make sure her airway is open. The ambulance is on its way." "Cynthia look at mommy, I don't know what to do, Cynthia stay with me, oh my God." The operator asked, "Is there anything coming out of her mouth?" "Yes, she's got some kind of foam, it's a pinkish colour." "Okay, put her on her side, the ambulance is on its way alright, they'll be there very shortly okay." "Okay." Click.

There I was, holding my daughter, talking to her, not knowing what to do, I felt so alone, so helpless. My daughter was lying on the kitchen floor, her legs bent totally backward from the fall, foaming at the mouth, moaning, and breathing very heavily making those strange noises, not able to answer me. I was on my knees, my phone in my hand but nobody at the other end.

It seemed like an eternity until I saw the ambulance arrive. Nothing seemed real. I answered the door and there stood two paramedics and four firefighters. The paramedics went to Cynthia, asking me questions, taking her blood pressure. They sat her up and asked her if she could stand up. She made the motion of standing up, however they had to carry her to the stretcher, which had been left outside. What the Hell had just happened? I phoned her father and told him what I knew. The paramedics asked me if I wanted to ride with them to the hospital, but I told them that I would follow in my car. I have no idea why I decided to drive other than I thought that I would need a car to bring Cynthia home later. I ran upstairs frazzled wondering what I needed, walking around in circles. I followed the ambulance, it was cold and raining. I met them at the emergency doors and as they brought her in I went to the front desk and registered her. After completing the paperwork like I had done just a few nights ago, I sat alone in that waiting room, with tears rolling down my cheeks, and waited for someone to tell me what was wrong with my daughter.

The hospital PA announcement blared: "Code Blue in the emergency room, Code Blue in the emergency room." Cynthia's father, Al, arrived and I summarized for him what had happened to this point. A nurse came out and showed us to a room. As we walked towards the room, I could see Cynthia's plaid pyjama pants and her burgundy T-shirt sticking out of the curtains. A few minutes later, the doctor-in-charge came in, closed the door, and sat down. That couldn't be good. He sat in front of us and very calmly said, "Cynthia has a problem breathing, she had a cardiac arrest for a few seconds, she's doing okay for now, I'll come back in a few minutes and tell you what we're going to do," and he left.

I sat on a couch and held my head in my hands. Al stood up pretended to punch the wall. We looked at each other, not understanding what was going on. Everything was surreal. We were both crying, trying to hold on, trying to be strong. I got up and looked out the window where I could see her feet still sticking out of the curtains. Suddenly, we heard: "Code Blue in the emergency room, Code Blue in the emergency room." The first Code Blue had been for my daughter, and now I hoped that this Code Blue was for someone else; it couldn't be for her again. I watched in disbelief as more and more nurses and doctors rushed through those curtains and worked to revive her. I watched as her lifeless legs jumped every time she received a jolt from the defibrillator paddles.

A few minutes later the doctor came in and gave us the news: "Cynthia had another cardiac arrest, we don't know why, we have called Toronto Sick Kids Hospital and we're arranging to send her there. They have the best care for her. We're arranging for transportation. As soon as they arrive we'll transfer her there."

What the Hell do I say to that? How do I wrap my head around what I've just witnessed, what I've just heard? What's going on? Was this real? I couldn't grasp what was going on. There I stood, feeling powerless and helpless, staring at my daughter's feet. Her dad grabbed his head with both hands in disbelief. This was my perfectly healthy rugby player laying there. Fuck!- What the Hell? – Have you felt so powerless, helpless that you feel sick? I froze, I couldn't believe what I was seeing, crying, standing there with a blank look on my face. I was like a zombie.

The doctor came in and told us we could go to Cynthia, to be close to her, to talk to her, and to stay with her. At the time I thought it was to comfort her. Looking back, I realized that they probably didn't think she was going to make it. Even though she looked okay, she didn't respond when we spoke to her. The staff would repeat that our daughter was very sick, yet nobody could tell us what was wrong with her, nobody knew.

About 20 minutes later, the ambulance from Sick Kids arrived and Cynthia was transferred by stretcher to it. The Ajax staff supplied a summary of the event to the three-person ambulance team, and we were ready to go.

The doctor suggested that one of us should ride with Cynthia in the ambulance. Al and I looked at each other and we decided that I would go. Al quickly asked me if I needed anything from my home and I answered, "Yes, I need my medicine and a warm sweater." I was freezing, I guess from all the emotions, and then I asked him to make sure to bring Cynthia's bear. "Bear" is Cynthia's teddy bear and she has had him since she was two years old. "Bear" knows all of Cynthia's secrets, all her sad and happy moments. It was important for me that she had him at her side for when she woke up.

CHAPTER 3
CCU—CRITICAL CARE UNIT

HERE I AM SITTING beside this tall, bald fellow. It was 5 am on May 21, and my daughter was in the back with two paramedics, doing their best to keep her alive, fighting for her life. The sun was rising, and the roads were deserted. The ambulance raced to reach Toronto Sick Kids Hospital, as quickly as possible. Tears were rolling down my cheeks, and I was trying to dry them off discreetly. The driver passed me a box of tissues and asked, "Do you have other children?" I replied, "Yes, I have a beautiful 14 year old daughter, her name is Samantha, she's at a friend's cottage this weekend." He responded, "I have two kids the same age as yours." I stared out the window, trying to remember the route he was taking so that I would know how to get there afterwards. Why? I have no clue.

He pulled the ambulance up to the entrance to Emergency. I got out and went to the back doors of the ambulance, not sure what to do. They unloaded Cynthia, while one paramedic continued to use a pump to help her to breathe. She did not look well. The four of us rushed Cynthia down hospital hallways, through a glass overpass, to finally reach the Intensive Care Unit. The paramedics asked me to take a seat in the hallway a few feet away from Cynthia's room.

As I sat there, in front of the nursing station, I was thinking how nice it was of them to let me stay so close to her. Flooding into Cynthia's room were doctors, nurses, and one machine after another.

They were ready for her, no fooling around, everyone seemed on a mission. One nurse stopped and asked me, "Are you Mom?"

I replied, "Yes." She asked, "Do you need anything, do you want a juice?" I answered, "No thanks, I'm fine just take care of my daughter." She replied, "We will, you'll see a lot of people going in and out of her room, we're getting her set up. Once we're done you'll be able to go in and see her. It might take a little time but you'll see her as soon as we're done. All right? You're sure you don't want anything?" "No thanks," I said.

I registered Cynthia, and her dad arrived shortly afterwards. We were taken to a Family Room. The room was small with a window overlooking the glass overpass that I had raced through earlier. There was a loveseat, a couple of chairs, a table, and a phone. It is a private room used by families to meet with the doctors caring for their loved ones. A nurse brought us some juice and cookies. Honestly, eating was the last thing on my mind, but we were told we needed to take care of ourselves and to eat to keep our strength up.

Finally I could see my daughter. They warned me that she was hooked to a lot of machines, that it might be overwhelming, but that she needed all of them. As I walked into the room, I saw how many people were around her. Doctors, nurses, at this point I knew nothing. We were introduced to Darcy, the nurse-in-charge. She was a friendly, young woman with brown curly hair and a beautiful smile. She made me feel welcome and managed to calm my fears. The ICU staff at Sick Kids made me feel like Cynthia was in good hands. They took the time to explain, to the best of their knowledge, what was going on and what they were doing for Cynthia.

There were so many machines around Cynthia, stuff that I had never seen before. She had tubes coming in and out from everywhere, her neck, her mouth, her nose, her leg, and her arms. I went to her bedside, kissed her forehead, held her lifeless hand, told her I loved her, and asked God to help her.

Many people from many different teams were introduced to us, and all said the same: "Don't worry about remembering the names, it's okay."

I felt numb and confused, yet I had so many things running through my mind. Will my child survive? Will she be like before?

Will she be brain damaged in any way? Would it be fair to want her back or ask for her back no matter what her disability? I would have given up everything, if I could just get her back.

I returned to the Family Room, and the doctor-in-charge, Dr. Peter Cox, bless him, joined us. He was the doctor that Ajax hospital had been communicating with when it all happened. He explained what he and his team had done for Cynthia. His team had hooked Cynthia to an ECMO machine, a heart and lung machine. The ECMO machine would take the blue blood out, process it, reoxygenate it, and then return it to Cynthia. To do this they had inserted a tube through her neck, which took the blue blood out, and had inserted another tube into her left leg for the processed blood to return. Normally, both tubes would have been inserted into the neck, however, because of Cynthia's age, the risk of a stroke was too great.

They had no idea what caused her medical crisis, but they were leaning toward a virus. They told me that sometimes viruses attack as fast as they leave. They were honest about it; they said maybe we would never know.

I was asked to provide details on what happened at home. I tried to answer the questions as completely as I could, determined not to leave anything out. I also gave them all the meds Cynthia had been taking. I was asked: Does she smoke? Does she drink? Has she gone out of the country in the last few months? Is she allergic to any meds? Any history of heart failure in the family? Any death due to heart complications? Did Cynthia have siblings? When I answered yes to the last question, I was told to have her sister brought to the hospital as soon as possible because at that point they weren't sure which way it was going to go.

CHAPTER 4
SAM

"HELLO," ANSWERED SAM. "HEY Sam, it's Mommy." "Hi Mommy," replied Sam. I was so happy to hear her voice and I tried to stay as calm and normal sounding as possible. "I tried calling you a few times but your phone was off," I said. "Oh I don't get service out here," she replied. "Hey, what are you doing?" I asked. "Well we're going to drive back to Toronto because it's raining out here and Haylea's dad wants to go, so." "Oh I see, well I'm calling you because Cynthia is really sick, I had to take her to the hospital and I want you to come here, so, because I'm at the hospital with your dad, your uncle Derek, will wait for you at home and he'll drive you here, okay?" "What's wrong with her? Is she okay?" Sam asked. "We don't know yet, so I'll see you in a bit okay?" "Okay." "I love you I'll see you soon, bye baby." "Love you too bye Mommy."

Sam, Cynthia's younger sister, was 14 years old at the time, a petite-framed girl, with long blond hair and green eyes. She has always been very happy-go-lucky and full of energy. She loved cheerleading and hanging out with her wide circle of friends. Always a social butterfly, her cellphone and MSN were big parts of her life. As often happens with two siblings, she's very different from her sister.

Sam was out of town when all this happened. She was vacationing at a friend's cottage 1½ hours from Toronto. I wanted her here so badly, and yet she was so far away. In the end, it gave me more time to think of how I would explain to her what was happening. A few hours later, Sam finally got to the hospital. I met her at the elevator with her dad; she was holding a Slurpee cup, holding flowers that she had picked for her sister, where I have no idea, but that's Sam. We walked to a window and sat on a bench. We sat and told Sam that Cynthia was very sick and that she was hooked to a lot of machines that were keeping her alive. Sam keeps most of her feeling inside, which I admit, sometimes scares me. She tried to keep it in but I saw two big tears roll down her soft cheeks. I gave her a big hug and asked her if she wanted to see her sister. At first she answered no, but I suggested that she should and promised her dad and I would go with her.

I held Sam as we walked in; I wasn't sure how she was going to react. I brought her to Cynthia's bedside and told her that she could hold Cynthia's hand and talk to her, and that Cynthia could hear us. At first she didn't want to but slowly and softly she held Cynthia's fingers, and cried while clinging to "Favory," her blanky. It was the only thing, at that point, which could comfort her. Like me, it didn't seem real to her. I'm not sure if Sam understood how seriously ill her sister was. It was probably better that way.

CHAPTER 5
THE WAIT

"YOU KNOW WHAT MIGHT be good? If you made Cynthia a poster with pictures of her family and friends," said Ruth. "That's a great idea, we'll ask Sam to work on that, thanks Ruth," I replied.

Ruth was the new nurse that was caring for Cynthia. You see unlike I thought you are assigned a new nurse every 12 hours, that's the length of their shift. What do I know? At that point not much. Never been in hospitals for a long period of time before. Some nurses care, some are there for the money, I guess like any work environment, but Ruth seemed like a very nice person, who kept me in reality. Ruth took the time to talk with me, explain what was going on, what she was doing, and also reminded me that my daughter was a very, very sick girl. She was a wise person to tell me that when I talked to my youngest daughter I should never say that everything would be alright, because nobody knew. "Keep it real," she said to me. Most nurses talked to Cynthia as they changed her dressing, or when they took blood. It was something I had never thought of, but of course, the patient needed to be told what was happening to them.

The next few days would determine if Cynthia would survive. Dr. Cox, the emergency doctor that had taken over when we arrived, sat with us and told us that on average a patient can stay hooked to an ECMO machine for only a certain amount of time, up to a maximum of a week. In the meantime, they were looking for different alternatives, perhaps a heart transplant, but they would do everything they could before they took that route. My mind raced: Would there be one available if she needed one? Would her body accept this new heart or reject it? At the same time, they noticed that her blood wasn't flowing properly to both atriums; that the reoxygenated blood was only going into one atrium of her heart, which caused the atrium to balloon. Cynthia would need a procedure to correct the blood flow to both atriums. This was overwhelming, to say the least, with lots of information coming at me at once, again. Dr. Cox proceeded to draw a picture of Cynthia's heart, which helped me to understand the problem she faced. They needed to make a "hole" between both atriums to help the blood flow. This hole would remain there; he mentioned that many people walk around with such a thing. There were so many questions going through my mind once more. He explained the risks, because there are always risks. It was going to be quite the process. Cynthia was hooked to so much equipment that it would take them one hour to prep her for the procedure, one hour for the actual procedure, and another hour to return her to her room, if everything went well. Each machine was staffed to ensure that nothing would come unhooked or tangled. They needed parent approval, but at this point it needed to be done and her dad and I signed the papers.

As I prayed that everything would be okay, my mind kept running through the whys, hows, and what ifs. I told God that I wouldn't ask Him for anything else for the rest of my life, just please make my daughter better. Sam and I huddled together and waited in the ICU parent waiting room—a room that we grew to know way too well. It was a fairly large room, divided into four different family areas. The room was furnished with golden faux leather couches, side tables with lamps, coffee tables, and a huge fish tank standing in one corner, donated by a family who had spent, I imagine, many hours also in that room. At the entrance to this room was a small white desk with a chair and a phone. Each time before we could visit Cynthia, we had to call the main ICU desk to ask if this was a good time and then receive the nurse's permission. Sam laid with me on the couch holding on to her blanket. We waited.

The procedure took 4½ hours; everything went well according to the doctors. An hour or so later Sam and I were told that we could see her. She looked the same, peaceful, yet still hooked to machines. I sat beside her thinking that a week ago she had been perfectly healthy and now she had almost been taken away from us forever. She couldn't breathe on her own, she couldn't talk to me. She could see me, and answer me by a nod or a squeeze of my fingers. I was happy to be there, to have her all to myself for the first time since this ordeal started. I knew I was being selfish but I needed that time with her. I was glad that I had the chance to communicate with her once more. Every little moment that I had alone with her I cherished. Nothing seemed to matter as much. For when it really came down to it, all I cared about were my daughters. I asked God for my daughter back. I promised to never feel sorry for myself as long as I had her. I have always been a strong believer that everything happened for a reason, yet I knew God would decide her destiny. It is said that He doesn't give you more than you can handle; this time it was a pretty big one if you ask me.

Cynthia had finally settled around 11:30 pm, considered early in her everyday life. We were at the end of the fourth day. Due to the seriousness of Cynthia's condition, Sam and I slept in a room the nurses had provided us with so we could remain close. I said my prayers for Cynthia that night with Sam, in French, like I used to do with them when they were little. Funny enough that the girls don't speak fluent French, but they know their prayers in French. I also thanked Him for giving us the beautiful gift of communicating with Cynthia today and to give her strength and determination to keep fighting. We both closed our eyes hoping to see Cynthia the next day.

CHAPTER 6
SICK KIDS

SATURDAY, MAY 27 ARRIVED, 24 hours since the procedure, and everything looked good. Cynthia was stable, although they were still monitoring her closely. I was concerned that Cynthia's seven-day time limit on the ECMO machine was approaching and I was feeling incredible stress. There was a respiratory technician guarding that machine around the clock. They were looking for blood clots, ensuring that there was always sufficient blood flow. All I could do was hope that they knew what they were doing.

Today was the day that they would lower the function of the ECMO machine to see how much of Cynthia's heart could function on its own. Unfortunately it didn't go as well as the doctors had hoped. However, they would try it again in a couple of days. Cynthia had many IVs and the lines had to cleaned, changed, replenished with meds, otherwise the machines would beep constantly until someone looked after it. Every time those machines beeped, I felt panic and wished for someone to hurry and do something.

By this time I had met Diane, the social worker for the ICU unit. Diane reminded me of Reese Witherspoon, blond, same shaped face, colourful dresser, nice smile. She offered moral support, answered my work-related questions, and guided me through my shock. Diane would come around everyday and made sure that we were okay.

Sick Kids is a very special hospital in the heart of Toronto. It's the premier hospital for children in North America. It is also a teaching hospital where doctors in training come to do their residency. Sick Kids has eight floors, and each floor has its specialty. The 2nd floor is for the CCU, ICU, and operating rooms.

The 4th floor is for general pediatrics, the 7th floor is for cardiac patients, and the 8th floor is for terminally ill children. There are six glass elevators, which the children love to ride. The walls of each floor have handpainted cartoon characters familiar to the children, such as Elmo, Big Bird, Dora, and Snoopy. The main floor is like a mini city, with a Tim Hortons, Harvey's, Shoppers Drug Mart, Roots, four restaurants, sitting areas, and beautiful fountains. Sick Kids is the only hospital downtown Toronto with a helicopter pad. It is situated amongst 3 other hospital which all linked underground to each other. Sick Kids is approximately 65 km from our house in Whitby, so 1 travel time.

If Cynthia had to be hospitalized, this certainly was the hospital to be in. I was told by Dr. Cox that had Cynthia been 18 years old, she probably would have died. Sick Kids is a childrens hospital and only accepts patients under the age of 18; she was three weeks shy of her 18th birthday when she arrived at Sick Kids.

CHAPTER 7
MORE PROCEDURES

"CAN YOU FEEL THIS?" asked the doctor. Cynthia nodded no. "Can you feel this?" Another no. She couldn't feel a thing, only on her frail face. That's when we realize that she couldn't feel anything. Cynthia had many tests done, such as MRIs and Cat scans, to try to understand what exactly she had. A few days after the first trial to take her off the ECMO machine, they tried again and this time Cynthia's own heart took over at 50-percent capacity. Success! They decided that no heart transplant would be required and they would disconnect her from the ECMO machine. That was scary for me. Nevertheless they did and her heart grew stronger.

Cynthia graduated from the Coronary Care Unit to the Intensive Care Unit, one step closer to a regular floor. That was amazing news, scary but great. There were, however, more complications appearing. Cynthia's left leg started to swell. They had been monitoring it for a while, and it seemed that the blood was not flowing properly. Unfortunately, they discovered that Cynthia had developed a blood clot in her left leg while she had been hooked to the ECMO machine. The doctors decided that surgery was necessary to insert an IVC filter, which would block any blood clot from travelling through the hole in her heart or to her brain. Once in place the filter would open up like an umbrella. There was a risk that pieces of the filter could break off or that the clot could be so big that it would actually stop the blood flow. Even with the risks involved, there was no other option. It was a temporary filter good for 100 days. Cynthia came out of surgery, with the filter in place, and I thought we were our way to recovery.

Cynthia complained that her vision was blurry; she would ask us to wipe her eyes, but it didn't really help because her sight had deteriorated. A big concern for Cynthia was her stomach. Anything she ate would go right through her. She was put on a diet to constipate her, we tried many things, unfortunately to this day she has chronic diarrhea. Sometimes I would change her diaper 30 times a day. Cynthia needed to be catheterized and changed often in a day. GBS was what they diagnosed her to have, affected her entire neuro system, which also included her digestive system. The esophagus wasn't working properly and foam would come up. To this day nobody seems to know what it is. I pretty much became a nurse. My days were full and exhausting but I needed to do something with myself. If my mommy powers weren't working anymore at least I could take care of her.

The next thing that GBS affected was her skin. Her entire body shed its skin, as if sunburned. It started with her arms and legs, moved to her hands, and then her feet. She also lost a fair amount of hair. For every stroke of the hairbrush, a huge amount of her hair would come with it. At the beginning I tried to hide it from her, but soon she couldn't help but notice. Bed sores were another complication. We needed to stop them from getting worse. She had one at the back of her head, on her heels, her bottom, and on the back of her left calf. To prevent future breakage, Cynthia was moved every three hours. She wore inflatable booties to keep her heel of the had surface of the bed. Cynthia also went through a nightmare stage. She was being weaned off the morphine, which had been used to sedate her while hooked to the ECMO machine, but now the withdrawal was causing delusions and nightmares: spiders on the wall and rain in the room.

Since Cynthia was having so many problems with her stomach, I asked if she could have tests done to see if there was anything abnormal going on. The X-ray showed that there was something wrong. Originally, when the first X-ray was done, they had thought that her shirt had created a shadow on the film. After the second X-ray, the same shadow appeared. They finally determined that two pieces of the IVC filter had broken off, one piece lodged in her heart and the other one in her lung. Yep, it could only happen to us. Anyway that's how I felt. They debated the risks and decided that it would be too risky to operate on the heart. Overtime the muscle of the heart would work around it. They did, however, remove the remainder of the filter to ensure that no other pieces would break off. We were back to square one: back in the operating room for another filter. This wasn't the cause of the stomach issue, however not asking to have the X-ray done, would we ever have found out?

We were introduced to the physiotherapy team and Cynthia began her first session. The plan was to gently shake her in order to loosen the phlegm and then suction it. The phlegm build up was from all the tubs that kept her alive. First they turn off the machine that would help her breath which made an annoying beeping sound when it was turned off. They needed to disconnect it in order to do the physio exercise. As they were doing this, Cynthia went into a seizure. I was watching a terrifying repeat of the seizure she had suffered at home. "Cynthia, are you okay? Cynthia, answer me? I begged. The nurse pushed the bell for Code Blue and about five doctors came out of nowhere. I was in the corner of the room crying, holding my head with both of hands, saying to myself this could not be happening again. Then she was back. Cynthia told me later: "You know Mom I could hear you but I couldn't talk. I saw the light at the end of the tunnel, I saw my entire life, and I had to decide which way I was going." From that day on she was scared to go to sleep, scared that she wouldn't wake up, or if she did fall asleep, she would wake up totally scared and gasping for air.

Later that day, after her seizure, she was able to lift her arms all by herself. We were astonished. What had just happened? Would the rest of her body be able to move too? With any small step of success we would encounter a huge setback.

CHAPTER 8
18TH BIRTHDAY

CYNTHIA'S 18TH BIRTHDAY WAS coming and we were told that she would be moved to the 4th floor, the cardiac floor. Chances looked good that she would spend her birthday in a regular hospital room with family and friends allowed to visit. Except for immediate family, visitors are not allowed in the CCU or ICU. Cynthia was hoping to be moved so that she could spend her 18th birthday surrounded by her family and friends.

For example, her uncle Derek was not allowed to see her, yet he sat outside every time he came and looked up at her window and spoke to her from out there, outside sitting on a bench facing her room. Others would come and visit with us in the waiting room even though they knew they couldn't go in to see her.

"Happy Birthday Cynthia," I said entering her ICU room. Today was her 18th birthday. Who could have imagined this birthday in hospital? We were celebrating two things, her birthday and her high school graduation. I asked the nurse, "Did you hear anything on when she'll be moving upstairs." "We're waiting for confirmation. They're not sure if she should go to the 4th or 7th floor," the nurse said. "Ok, so what does it mean?" I asked. "They need to decide if she is still a cardiac patient or if she is now considered pediatric," she answered. "Bureaucracy exists everywhere, well let us know because Cynthia is getting anxious to be in her room, today being her birthday," I said. "I understand, I'll do my best," she responded. The day went on and the nurse finally came back and announced, "Cynthia won't be moving upstairs today." That broke my heart, she was looking so forward to it, to be able to see everyone. But the nurse added, "We can transfer her into her previous room in CCU so you can have a little party for her, close the door and have everyone in the room with her." "That sounds good," I said, "Thanks for trying to make this birthday special for her."

We moved fast. Sam and I moved her belongings into the new room. We decorated the room, and her cousins, Eden and Melanie, had made a huge birthday banner that Sam and I hung. Cynthia's grandmother Barber had made her a banana cake and a carrot cake. The staff at Sick Kids sent a huge cake with plates and forks. We had the radio playing to create a non-hospital ambiance. Cynthia looked good, her hair was French-braided, and she had a big smile on her face.

There were a lot of special birthday wishes in that room: Corey, her boyfriend, Justin, Corey's best friend and also Cynthia's friend, her father and her grandparents, the Barbers, Sam, and me. A few nurses and doctors dropped in too. We tried to make it the best party that we could considering the circumstances. Everyone knew it was a big birthday and that it sucked being in here. Diane, the social worker, came in with a big brown bag decorated by hand with a felt maker. The hospital staff had given Cynthia a stuffed frog, a Blockbuster gift card, and a game. I was touched to see how much they cared. It had been a great birthday but as the afternoon wore on she grew very tired from the excitement of it all.

My birthday is a few days after hers. Cynthia made me wear a homemade badge that announced: "It's my birthday today." I just had to wear it for her.

CHAPTER 9
NEW HOME

"You'll be going on 7D," a nurse tells us. Finally, we had graduated from CCU to ICU to a regular room. I remember the day that I actually said to another mother waiting to take the elevator on the 2nd floor: "I can't wait for the day that I'll be taking my daughter to another floor." At the time, that day seemed so far away and now it was here. Cynthia's room overlooked the restaurant area; it had a couch that could be turned into a cot, and a full bathroom with all the accessories required to aid someone with needs. As the days went I was more and more involved with Cynthia's care. I would get there early in the morning and leave around 7 at night. Cynthia had more bad days than good days. Her stomach problem wasn't getting any better. Nothing would stay down. We joked that all the vomiting that she had suffered during June and July resulted in some nice abs.

Very special people work at Sick Kids. Marlene, Sandra, and Tamara, three exceptional nurses that cared for Cynthia, still keep in touch with us. More than a patient/nurse relationship was created; these women touched our lives. Tuesdays were special to us as we looked forward to our special visitor. Her name was Choola, a volunteer who dressed as a clown and brought smiles to sick children. Cynthia created a very special relationship with Choola. She knew exactly what to do to make Cynthia smile. They created such a bond that Cynthia became Choola's "manager." Choola would decorate Cynthia's door window with drawing, she would tattoo Cynthia's arm, she would pretend playing rock songs with her broom just to make us laugh. Once Choola said: "If you're in, you're in and if you out, you're out." And that stayed with us. The first time I met Choola she was in an elevator, dressed in her costume of green polka dot dress, white stockings, pink bow in her hair, and duster in hand. By the time she left the elevator, everyone, adults included, had a smile. That was the power of Choola!

I was naïve back then. I thought doctors knew it all, but I realized soon enough that medicine is for the most part a guessing game. When did I realize this? When Cynthia was on 15 different meds for one dosage 3 times a day and it wasn't making any difference on her situation. She had had enough; none of them seemed to decrease the pain or make anything better. That's when she decided to eliminate many of them, and she didn't get any worse. With all the complications throughout our journey at Sick Kids, her leg problems really started to concern many. Dr. Oreopolous and his team arrived from Toronto General Hospital to explain what was happening to Cynthia's swollen left leg this time.

He explained that when the ECMO tube was removed from her leg, the stitching to close the main artery hadn't healed properly. The second operation to fix it, unfortunately didn't take either and her body rejected the piece. I still felt that the artery hadn't been closed properly. It was time to operate for the third time. We had two options: use part of Cynthia's right leg artery and implant it into the left, risking the function of her right leg, or to use a cadaver's artery. Cynthia was transferred to Toronto General so Dr. Oreopolous could operate on Cynthia's leg.

The entire journey was emotional for many different reasons. We were leaving Sick Kids, a hospital and staff that we were very familiar with, to an unknown. Because she was coming from Sick Kids, Cynthia was admitted to a private room. I had to double check that we wouldn't be charged; my insurance didn't cover a private room and I hadn't been at work for the last few months. Cynthia was started on a treatment of GBS meds called IVIG, intravenous immunoglobulin, which made her very sick the entire time we were there. Unfortunately, she was too weak for the surgery to repair the aneurysm in her left leg and she was returned to Sick Kids. That's an operation that we postponed.

For the next few weeks she worked on physio: standing up for one minute, stretching, and using the hated tilt table for balance issues. Unable to transfer on her own, I would use the lift to move her to a wheelchair and take her out of her room. Even though I could only take her out for 20 minutes at a time—that's all she could tolerate—she enjoyed the fresh air and sunshine. Cynthia had reached a plateau in her recovery and we needed to look at the next step.

CHAPTER 10
DIAGNOSED—GUILLAIN-BARRE SYNDROME

"Can you feel this?" they asked Cynthia. "No," she said. "This?" "No." These types of questions continued at every visit with the neurology team, led by Dr. Brenda Banwell of Sick Kids Hospital. Even though Cynthia had been at Sick Kids for 2½ months and her discharge was coming soon, we still didn't have a diagnosis. There was the possibility that it was Guillain-Barré Syndrome, better known as GBS. Cynthia's symptoms were similar; however, she had far more complications than a typical GBS sufferer.

After much testing, poking, probing, and researching, Dr. Banwell diagnosed Cynthia with non-typical GBS.

What are the symptoms of GBS and what is it?
Guillain-Barré Syndrome is a disorder in which the body's immune system attacks part of the peripheral nervous system. The first symptoms of this disorder include varying degrees of weakness or tingling sensations in the legs. In many instances the weakness and abnormal sensations spread to the arms and upper body. These symptoms can increase in intensity until certain muscles cannot be used at all and, when severe, the patient is almost totally paralyzed. In these cases the disorder is life threatening—potentially interfering with breathing and, at times, with blood pressure or heart rate—and is considered a medical emergency.

Such a patient is often put on a respirator to assist with breathing and is watched closely for problems such as an abnormal heart beat, infections, blood clots, and high or low blood pressure. Most patients, however, recover from even the most severe cases of Guillain-Barré Syndrome, although some continue to have a certain degree of weakness.

Guillain-Barré Syndrome can affect anybody. It can strike at any age and both sexes are equally prone to the disorder. GBS is rare, however, afflicting only about one person in 100,000. Usually Guillain-Barré occurs a few days or weeks after the patient has had symptoms of a respiratory or gastrointestinal viral infection. Occasionally surgery or vaccinations will trigger the syndrome.

After the first clinical manifestations of the disease, the symptoms can progress over the course of hours, days, or weeks. Most people reach the stage of greatest weakness within the first two weeks after symptoms appear, and by the third week of the illness 90 percent of all patients are at their weakest.

What causes Guillain-Barré Syndrome?

No one yet knows why Guillain-Barré—which is not contagious—strikes some people and not others. Nor does anyone know exactly what sets the disease in motion.

What scientists do know is that the body's immune system begins to attack the body itself, causing what is known as an autoimmune disease. Usually the cells of the immune system attack only foreign material and invading organisms. In Guillain-Barré Syndrome, however, the immune system starts to destroy the myelin sheath that surrounds the axons of many peripheral nerves, or even the axons themselves (axons are long, thin extensions of the nerve cells; they carry nerve signals). The myelin sheath surrounding the axon speeds up the transmission of nerve signals and allows the transmission of signals over long distances.

In diseases in which the peripheral nerves' myelin sheaths are injured or degraded, the nerves cannot transmit signals efficiently. That is why the muscles begin to lose their ability to respond to the brain's commands, commands that must be carried through the nerve network. The brain also receives fewer sensory signals from the rest of the body, resulting in an inability to feel textures, heat, pain, and other sensations. Alternately, the brain may receive inappropriate signals that result in tingling, "crawling-skin," or painful sensations. Because the signals to and from the arms and legs must travel the longest distances they are most vulnerable to interruption. Therefore, muscle weakness and tingling sensations usually first appear in the hands and feet and progress upwards.

When Guillain-Barré is preceded by a viral or bacterial infection, it is possible that the virus has changed the nature of cells in the nervous system so that the immune system treats them as foreign cells. It is also possible that the virus makes the immune system itself less discriminating about what cells it recognizes as its own, allowing some of the immune cells, such as certain kinds of lymphocytes and macrophages, to attack the myelin. Sensitized T lymphocytes cooperate with B lymphocytes to produce antibodies against components of the myelin sheath and may contribute to destruction of the myelin. Scientists are investigating these and other possibilities to understand why the immune system goes awry in Guillain-Barré Syndrome and other autoimmune diseases. The cause and course of Guillain-Barré Syndrome is an active area of neurological investigation, incorporating the cooperative efforts of neurological scientists, immunologists, and virologists.

How is Guillain-Barré treated?

There is no known cure for Guillain-Barré Syndrome. However, there are therapies that lessen the severity of the illness and accelerate the recovery in most patients. There are also a number of ways to treat the complications of the disease.

Currently, plasma exchange (sometimes called plasmapheresis) and high-dose immunoglobulin therapy are used. Both of them are equally effective, but immunoglobulin is easier to administer. Plasma exchange is a method by which whole blood is removed from the body and processed so that the red and white blood cells are separated from the plasma, or liquid portion of the blood. The blood cells are then returned to the patient without the plasma, which the body quickly replaces. Scientists still don't know exactly why plasma exchange works, but the technique seems to reduce the severity and duration of the Guillain-Barré episode. This may be because the plasma portion of the blood contains elements of the immune system that may be toxic to the myelin.

In high-dose immunoglobulin therapy, doctors give intravenous injections of the proteins that, in small quantities, the immune system uses naturally to attack invading organisms. Investigators have found that giving high doses of these immunoglobulins, derived from a pool of thousands of normal donors, to Guillain-Barré patients can lessen the immune attack on the nervous system. Investigators don't know why or how this works, although several hypotheses have been proposed.

The use of steroid hormones has also been tried as a way to reduce the severity of Guillain-Barré, but controlled clinical trials have demonstrated that this treatment not only is not effective but may even have a deleterious effect on the disease.

The most critical part of the treatment for this syndrome consists of keeping the patient's body functioning during recovery of the nervous system. This can sometimes require placing the patient on a respirator, a heart monitor, or other machines that assist body function. The need for this sophisticated machinery is one reason why Guillain-Barré Syndrome patients are usually treated in hospitals, often in an intensive care ward. In the hospital, doctors can also look for and treat the many problems that can afflict any paralyzed patient—complications such as pneumonia or bed sores.

Often, even before recovery begins, caregivers may be instructed to manually move the patient's limbs to help keep the muscles flexible and strong. Later, as the patient begins to recover limb control, physical therapy begins. Carefully planned clinical trials of new and experimental therapies are the key to improving the treatment of patients with Guillain-Barré Syndrome. Such clinical trials begin with the research of basic and clinical scientists who, working with clinicians, identify new approaches to treating patients with the disease.

What is the long-term outlook for those with Guillain-Barré Syndrome?

Guillain-Barré Syndrome can be a devastating disorder because of its sudden and unexpected onset. In addition, recovery is not necessarily quick. As noted above, patients usually reach the point of greatest weakness or paralysis days or weeks after the first symptoms occur. Symptoms then stabilize at this level for a period of days, weeks, or, sometimes, months. The recovery period may be as little as a few weeks or as long as a few years. About 30 percent of those with Guillain-Barré still have a residual weakness after three years. About 3 percent may suffer a relapse of muscle weakness and tingling sensations many years after the initial attack.

Guillain-Barré Syndrome patients face not only physical difficulties, but emotionally painful periods as well. It is often extremely difficult for patients to adjust to sudden paralysis and dependence on others for help with routine daily activities. Patients sometimes need psychological counselling to help them adapt.

What research is being done?

Scientists are concentrating on finding new treatments and refining existing ones. Scientists are also looking at the workings of the immune system to find which cells are responsible for beginning and carrying out the attack on the nervous system. The fact that so many cases of Guillain-Barré begin after a viral or bacterial infection suggests that certain characteristics of some viruses and bacteria may activate the immune system inappropriately. Investigators are searching for those characteristics. Certain proteins or peptides in viruses and bacteria may be the same as those found in myelin, and the generation of antibodies to neutralize the invading viruses or bacteria could trigger the attack on the myelin sheath. As noted previously, neurological scientists, immunologists, virologists, and pharmacologists are all working collaboratively to learn how to prevent this disorder and to make better therapies available when it strikes.

Adapted from "Guillain-Barré Syndrome Fact Sheet," NIH Publication No. 05-2902, National Institute of Neurological Disorders and Stroke.

CHAPTER 11
LYNDHURST REHABILITATION CENTRE

AFTER THREE MONTHS AT Sick Kids, Cynthia wanted to go home, she didn't want to hear of another place where she'd have to meet new staff, etc. Unfortunately, it wasn't an option at this time and staff from Lyndhurst Rehabilitation Centre visited us at Sick Kids. Social worker, Nick, and two physiotherapists, Jamie and Mel, answered our many questions. After what we had been through, it was very scary to think of my daughter at a facility that didn't have the same medical support as a hospital. I knew that once we left Sick Kids we wouldn't be accepted back. Now that she was 18, if she had a major setback she would be sent to another hospital, Sunnybrook or Toronto General, and no one would have a history of these last three months.

Cynthia arrived at Toronto's Lyndhurst Centre on August 16. Lyndhurst was constructed during World War Two to help wounded soldiers recover from their injuries. Lyndhurst was old, tired-looking, and under renovation. Cynthia's was in a four-person room, similar to a hospital ward, with curtains for dividers. Each patient had a desk and a pantry/wardrobe. Cynthia was lucky enough to have one of the two beds by the huge window. About 20 minutes after we arrived, another patient was admitted to the room. Her name was Diane and she had sat for six hours in a wheelchair on a train from Timmins, Ontario. We were given a tour of the facility: common areas for dining, physio, gym, occupational therapy area with a kitchen and all appliances that one would need to survive, a chapel (under construction), main hall with a pool table, and another room with a car, yes, a car. I couldn't understand why at first, but then it all made sense. Lyndhurst's purpose is to teach patients to become independent as much as possible before being sent home. The car is to teach them how to get in and out of a vehicle and also how to dismantle their wheelchair, to be self-sufficient. Each wing had a tiny laundry room for patients to wash their clothes, and also a TV room.

We were told that Cynthia would stay at Lyndhurst for about four months. We met Dr. McGilvery, the doctor assigned to Cynthia during her stay there. Melanie was Cynthia's physiotherapist, young, a very nice smile, a sweet person. Part of the physiotherapy was to learn how to transfer from bed to wheelchair, build muscle strength, relearn to walk, increase the upright position with the famous tilt table, use the stationary bike, and to walk using parallel bars for support. After a month or so of physiotherapy, Cynthia took her first steps holding on to the parallel bars. I was stunned, I was moved to tears. Abbie was Cynthia's occupational therapist and her focus was on improving Cynthia's small motor skills, relearning how to hold a spoon, picking up small screws, working on sensation. Many times the therapists would dip Cynthia's hand in warm wax, peel the wax off, and then by using a fork, ask Cynthia if she could feel the poking; the answer was always no. Physio and occupational therapy were each scheduled for one hour everyday.

In the first early days of her stay, Cynthia would have her meals in her room, but by the second week she started making her way to the dining room. Now came the socializing...something she hadn't done for a while. I was proud of her; she made some new acquaintances. Most of the patients were men or older women, but there were two younger girls, Michele who sang and played the piano beautifully and Fazila the oldest of five siblings. Everyone at Lyndhurst had a story. Every patient was in a wheelchair and I realized how fortunate I was that my daughter had a chance to walk again, unlike many of the others. Charlene was Cynthia's recreational therapist and she was in charge of reintegrating patients into everyday life by organizing various outings for the patients.

A week after we arrived, Cynthia was supplied an electric wheelchair. This made her feel independent for the first time in a long time. In record time she had that chair under control, although once she rammed it into a wall and totally scraped her hand. She looked at her hurt hand and in all seriousness, said to me, "Damn that must have hurt!" I had to laugh at how far we had come. Now we found some humour in the fact that Cynthia couldn't feel anything, and yes, she was right, it must have hurt!

Cynthia was doing better since arriving at Lyndhurst. She was finally diagnosed with being lactose intolerant, which explained some of her digestive troubles at Sick Kids. Little things like that gave me hope, that maybe someone knew what they were doing. She was put on a different med for her ongoing diarrhea, which made her feel confident to venture from her room. Things were looking up. As the days went by and because of Cynthia's hard work, we saw improvement. Her low blood pressure was still a major concern, but they were trying to find the right dosage to correct it.

I was counting down the days until I would have to return to work. I knew how fortunate I was to have been able to be with my daughter all this time but now I had to wean her off my everyday presence. Overtime, Cynthia was making more and more friends at Lyndhurst, still dealing with her everyday pain and discomfort, but I could see improvement. Thanksgiving was approaching and Cynthia still had no feeling or sensation anywhere but her face, but she showed great spirit.

CHAPTER 12
KEEPING THE SPIRIT

Trick or Treat! Halloween was approaching and in our house it was always a great celebration. It was two months from first arriving at Lyndhurst and five months from the start of our journey. Cynthia had the great idea to decorate her chair as a throne and she would be a queen for Halloween. Her friend, Fazila, would be the king. We used our occupational therapy time to make the costume. Using four poster-sized cardboard, we cut out the shape of a Victorian chair and decorated it with gold glitter. Her idea was grand and it turned out great. Wearing a crown and a red velvet cape she went around the centre, handing out candies to all the patients and their families. She even went out into the nearby community with her dad that night and trick or treated for candies of her own.

During her stay at Lyndhurst, Cynthia suffered numerous bladder infections and dehydration, to the point that twice she had to be sent to Sunnybrook Hospital for treatment. Christmas was coming, another favorite holiday for the family. With Cynthia's recurring infections, I had to keep our spirits up, not knowing when Cynthia would be discharged. To improve on the outlook of a sad Christmas at Lyndhurst, I decided to make Cynthia's occupational therapy more exciting with a Christmas project. I bought six little reindeer, fake snow, tiny Christmas lights, and Cynthia and I made decorations. I decided that if this year she couldn't actually decorate our house, the next best thing would be for her to help decorate Lyndhurst. So we did, we made six festive reindeer for the dining room. I think the people there appreciated our Christmas spirit and I was proud of what Cynthia had accomplished.

CHAPTER 13
DISCHARGE

"I'LL BE TAKING THE minutes at today's meeting," Charlene said. There we were, sitting at the table for what turned out to be our last family meeting at Lyndhurst. Since arriving at Lyndhurst, every family meeting consisted of one representative from each area of Cynthia's rehabilitation. Our last meeting included Dr. McGilvery, a social worker, an occupational, recreational, and physiotherapist, a pharmacist, a community access to care (CCAC) rep, her dad, and me. Cynthia's discharge date would be December 14. Two weeks from now and seven months from the start of our journey, Cynthia would be coming home to her sister Sam and me.

In the last month or so I had arranged to have the house renovated so that it was wheelchair accessible. The carpet was removed and replaced with hardwood to make the wheelchair easier to manouevre, and a stair glide was installed to allow Cynthia to get to her second-floor bedroom. This sounds easy but let me take you back a few weeks. I was told that in order to allow my daughter to come home I must have a list of physical changes made to my house so she could lead as normal of a life as possible. But there was a catch.

I looked at all the alternatives to get my daughter home... selling the house to find a one-level home, to extending the back of the house so that we wouldn't need an elevator or stair glide. I received very little help on what I could and could not do. Nevertheless, an amazing man, who I referred to earlier in this book as "Puck" the rugby coach, came to our rescue. His devotion and concern for us throughout this ordeal was commendable. I hope that everyone has the chance to come across their own

"Puck." He held fundraising events at Cynthia's high school, which helped to defray the cost of renovating our home.

Those funds helped pay for the wheelchair ramp, hardwood flooring, and also covered some of the cost of the wheelchair. You see, that's where the system failed us. I filed for funding, however, I was told it would take six months to a year for approval; in the meantime, I needed the funds to renovate my house so my daughter could come home. I was told that any money I spent prior to funding approval would not be reimbursed. I was told I could apply for funding yet it was a Catch-22 situation. Bless "Puck" and his extraordinary help.

Still very ill, Cynthia came home for good on December 14, with Corey and Sam waiting for her. I was happy, sad, scared, and many other emotions that day. I was happy to have my daughter home after these long seven months, sad because she was leaving behind the friends she had made at Lyndhurst, and scared of the many unknowns ahead of us.

CHAPTER 14
AS THE MONTHS PASS

TODAY IS NOVEMBER 12 and I'm on my way to Montreal for meetings. Many things have happened over the last year. Medically, Cynthia underwent another surgery in February on her leg to improve the blood flow. We've had many doctors' appointments over the last 10 months. Specialists in blood clots, blood pressure, GBS, and neurology all say the same thing: "With time and lots of physio." I've learned that medicine is sometimes practiced by trial and error. No one knows for certain and I'm not convinced to this day that they believe Cynthia has GBS. Her health has approved, although she still has a long way to go and at times wants to give up. Her digestive system hasn't come back yet, she still catheterizes herself, and sensation, other than to her face, hasn't come back. She continues to risk cross-medications, burns, low blood pressure, and bladder infections, which take over her entire body requiring many stays in hospital on antibiotic intravenous drips.

Cynthia has been involved in different activities with the Lyndhurst Centre. Charlene, the recreational therapist, stays in touch and gives Cynthia the opportunity to join various programs. She has enjoyed bucket water skiing, archery, canoeing, gliding, and bucket downhill skiing. We have adapted the best that we can to our new way of life. Cynthia went for pool physiotherapy, which helped her progress more than any other therapy to date.

One needs to keep a sense of humour to get through this; you don't really have a choice. I realize that life is too short and too unknown to worry about the silly stuff. I don't think Sam has totally accepted what happened to her sister and our family. She recently told me, "Do you realize that I have as much education as Cyn now?" And Cynthia declares, "Mom, do you realize that Sam has her driver's licence?" I guess in a perfect world the oldest paves the road for the youngest but for us it is different world.

CHAPTER 15
HOPE

TODAY IS JUNE 1, 2009, three years since our journey began, and I want to give you the latest update and show you that there is still hope not matter what has happened to you or your family. Still to this day, Cynthia has feeling only in her face, but in the last year, she has steadily progressed to where she is able to walk around the house and take the stairs up and down without use of a wheelchair or stair glide. Her social life has increased and she is slowly working on obtaining her Home Staging certificate. Her friends from high school still keep in touch and are great to her. Cynthia's weight is still a challenge at 97 pounds, and although she eats well it is still a struggle to put the weight back on. She will be turning 21 soon and it's time for the next step. She has applied for housing that is wheelchair accessible since she still uses a wheelchair when she is extremely fatigued or while shopping, etc. We finally took the wheelchair ramp down a few weeks ago since Cynthia hasn't needed it in the last year. We will donate the chair glide to someone that could make good use of it.

Cynthia's next medical appointment is with Dr. Hans, GBS specialist out of London, Ontario. We met Dr. Hans this past May at a GBS conference in Toronto. This conference was quite emotional for me; it was the first time I heard someone else tell "my story." I wasn't crazy after all...someone out there knew exactly what I was saying and going through. We are currently waiting for Dr. Banwell, Cynthia's neurologist at Sick Kids, to send all information regarding Cynthia's stay at Sick Kids to Dr. Hans for review. Dr. Hans will then give us a final second opinion.

Of course, I wish I had known of Dr. Hans before, but I suppose everything happens for a reason, sometimes you just don't know why.

From what we learned at the conference, Dr. Hans has helped many patients that were wrongly diagnosed and throughout her career has made a huge difference in many lives. She is a scientist who has devoted her life to GBS and CIDP (Chronic Inflammatory Demyelinating Polyneuropathy). She is nearing retirement and we are grateful and honoured that she has agreed to give us her medical opinion, even though she stated at the conference that Cynthia's case is one of the most complicated cases she has ever heard of. There is hope that Cynthia may get even better than she is now. And if not, then I will be continued to be thankful that my daughter can think, talk, walk, move, eat, laugh, and be who she is.

Sam is graduating from high school this month, and will be attending Niagara College in September, studying General Arts and Science: Acting for Film and Television. Sam is an amazing young woman and will do well in life in any field related to TV, radio, stage manager, etc.

I started a new job in January and love it. I have a special man in my life that gives me tremendous support everyday and treats me like a queen. He is very supportive of my girls and we enjoy life more and more everyday.

I hope this book has helped you understand a little more about GBS. Look for more answers to your unanswered questions. Keep pushing for what you believe is right for you and your family. Do not be scared to ask questions. Listen to your "little" voice; if it doesn't feel right, then it's not. Reach out to those you trust.

To those dealing with GBS, remember that you have to play the cards you were dealt, one way or another.

ACKNOWLEDGEMENTS

I WOULD LIKE TO extend my sincere thanks to everyone that supported me through this journey. I have met many wonderful people. Dr. Cox for saving my daughter's life, the nurses at Sick Kids, Ruth, Marlene, Sandra, Sarah and Tamara. Puck, for all the hard work he has done to help our family, from fund raising to renovation, visits at the hospital. My friends; Janice, Cindy, Sarah, Lynn, Lisa for going out of their way to help.

To my editor also taxi driver Erin, who took many hours of her busy day to drive Cynthia to her appointments, for the many long conversations that she had with Cynthia and editing my book.

Author Bio

Guylaine Fortier-Barber:

Born and raised in Victoriaville, Quebec, youngest of three girls, Guylaine made her life in Toronto when she was 18. She has two beautiful daughters. An energetic professional, she shares her experiences with a syndrome that few know about, to inspire others to find strength when feeling powerless, and to create awareness of Guillain-Barré Syndrome.